Keto Diet for Over 50

Your key to prove

age doesn't matter

Lucy Cooper

TABLE OF CONTENTS

Readers acknowledge that the author is not engaging in the rendering of legal, financial, medical or professional advice. The content within this book has been derived from various sources. Please consult a licensed professional before attempting any techniques outlined in this book. By reading this document, the reader agrees that under no circumstances is the author responsible for any losses, 5 direct or indirect, which are incurred as a result of the use of information contained within this document, including, but not limited to, — errors, omissions, or inaccuracies.

BREAKFAST

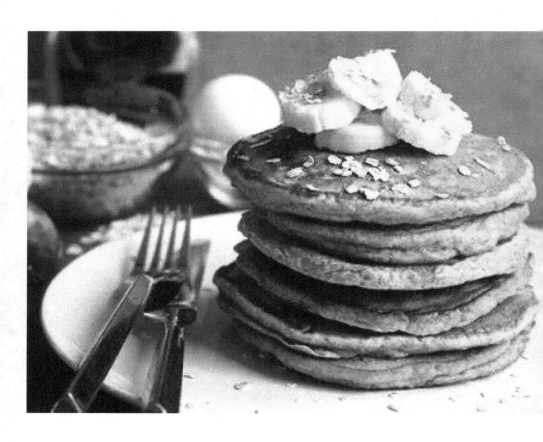

Easy Vanilla Granola

Servings: 6

Cooking Time: 1 Hour

Ingredients

- ½ cup hazelnuts, chopped
- 1 cup walnuts, chopped
- ⅓ cup flax meal
- ⅓ cup coconut milk
- ⅓ cup poppy seeds
- ⅓ cup pumpkin seeds
- 8 drops stevia
- ⅓ cup coconut oil, melted
- 1 ½ tsp vanilla paste
- 1 tsp ground cloves
- 1 tsp grated nutmeg
- 1 tsp lemon zest
- ⅓ cup water

Directions:

1. Set oven to 300° F. Line a parchment paper to a baking sheet. Combine all ingredients. Spread the mixture onto the baking sheet in an even layer. Bake for 55 minutes, as you stir at intervals of minutes. Let cool at room temperature.

Nutrition Info (Per Serving): Kcal 449; Fat: 44.9g, Net Carbs: 5.1g, Protein: 9.3g

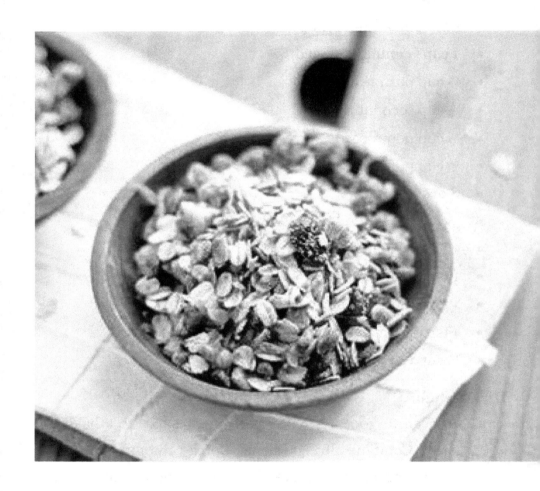

Cheese Omelet

Servings: 2

Cooking Time: 10 minutes

Ingredients

- 1.5 oz butter, unsalted
- 2 eggs
- 1 ounce shredded mozzarella cheese, full-fat
- Seasoning:
- ¼ tsp salt
- 1/8 tsp ground black pepper

Directions:

1. Take a medium bowl, crack eggs in it, whisk until blended and then whisk in half of the cheese, salt, and black pepper.
2. Take a frying pan, place it over medium heat, add butter and when it melts, pour in egg mixture, spread it evenly and let it cook for 2 minutes until set.
3. Switch heat to the low level, continue cooking for 2 minutes until thoroughly cooked, and then top with remaining cheese.
4. Fold the omelet, slide it to a plate, cut it in half, and then serve.

Nutrition Info: 275 Calories; 25.7 g Fats; 10.3 g Protein; 0.7 g Net Carb; 0 g Fiber;

Pancakes

Servings: 2

Cooking Time: 6 minutes

Ingredients

- ¼ cup almond flour
- 1 ½ tbsp unsalted butter
- 2 oz cream cheese, softened
- 2 eggs

Directions:

1. Take a bowl, crack eggs in it, whisk well until fluffy, and then whisk in flour and cream cheese until well combined.
2. Take a skillet pan, place it over medium heat, add butter and when it melts, drop pancake batter in four sections, spread it evenly, and cook for minutes per side until brown. Serve.

Nutrition Info: 166.8 Calories; 15 g Fats; 5.8 g Protein; 1.8 g Net Carb; 0.8 g Fiber

Egg Muffins with Bacon

Servings: 6

Cooking Time: 20 minutes

Ingredients

- 6 large eggs
- ½ cup cooked bacon, chopped
- ½ cup cheddar cheese, shredded
- salt and pepper, to taste
- ½ teaspoon dried basil
- ½ teaspoon dried oregano
- chives for garnish optional

Directions:

1. Preheat the oven to 350° F.
2. Whisk together the eggs, salt, pepper, dried basil and dried oregano. Mix well. Add the chopped bacon and shredded cheddar cheese. Stir.
3. Fill each muffin cup with the egg mixture. Bake for 15 minutes.
4. Garnish with chives and serve. Bon appetite!

Nutrition Info (Per Serving): 156 Calories; 12.8g Fat; 3.9g Carbs; 0.5g Fiber; 10g Protein

Cheese and Oregano Muffins

Servings: 6

Cooking Time: 25 minutes

Ingredients

- 2 tablespoons olive oil
- 1 egg
- 2 tablespoons parmesan cheese
- ½ teaspoon oregano, dried
- 1 cup almond flour
- ¼ teaspoon baking soda
- Salt and black pepper to the taste
- ½ cup of coconut milk
- 1 cup cheddar cheese, grated

Directions:

1. In a bowl, mix flour with oregano, salt, pepper, parmesan and baking soda and stir.
2. In another bowl, mix coconut milk with egg and olive oil and stir well.
3. Combine the 2 mixtures and whisk well.
4. Add cheddar cheese, stir, pour this a lined muffin tray, introduce in the oven at 350 degrees F for 25 minutes.
5. Leave your muffins to cool down for a few minutes, divide them between plates and serve.
6. Enjoy!

Nutrition Info: calories 160, fat 3, fiber 2, carbs 6, protein 10

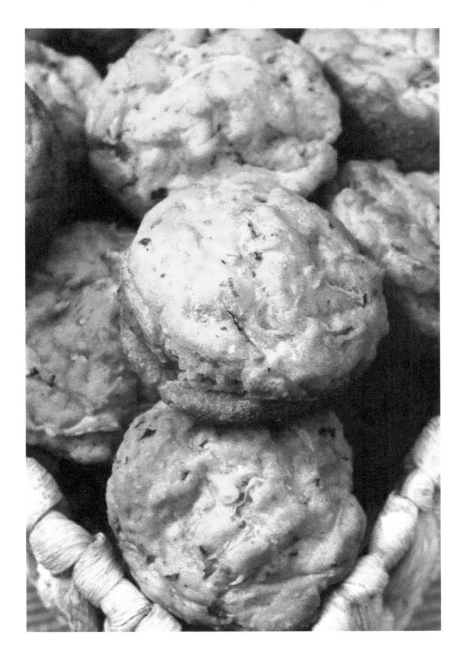

Crêpes with Lemon-buttery Syrup

Servings: 6

Cooking Time: 25 minutes

Ingredients

Crêpes:

- 6 ounces mascarpone cheese, softened
- 6 eggs
- 1 ½ tbsp granulated swerve
- ¼ cup almond flour
- 1 tsp baking soda
- 1 tsp baking powder

Syrup:

- ¾ cup of water
- 2 tbsp lemon juice
- 1 tbsp butter
- ¾ cup swerve, powdered
- 1 tbsp vanilla extract
- ½ tsp xanthan gum

Directions:

1. With the use of an electric mixer, mix all crepes ingredients until well incorporated.
2. Use melted butter to grease a frying pan and set over medium heat; cook the crepes until the edges start to

brown, about minutes. Flip over and cook the other side for a further 2 minutes; repeat the process with the remaining batter. Put the crepes on a plate.

3. In the same pan, mix swerve, butter and water; simmer for 6 minutes as you stir. Transfer the mixture to a blender together with a ¼ teaspoon of xanthan gum and vanilla extract and mix well. Place in the remaining xanthan gum, lemon juice, and allow to sit until the syrup is thick.

Nutrition Info (Per Serving): Kcal 243, Fat: 19.6g, Net Carbs: 5.5g, Protein: 11g

BRUNCH

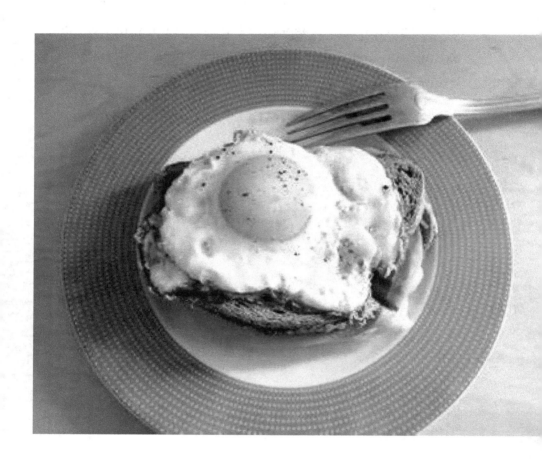

Ham and Emmental Eggs

Servings: 5

Cooking Time: 20 minutes

Ingredients

- 1 tbsp olive oil
- 4 slices ham, chopped
- ½ cup chives, chopped
- ½ cup broccoli, chopped
- 1 clove garlic, minced
- 1 tsp fines herbes
- ¼ cup vegetable broth
- 5 eggs
- 1 ½ cups Emmental cheese, shredded

Directions:

1. In a frying pan, warm oil. Add in ham and cook for 4 minutes, until brown and crispy; set aside.
2. Using the same pan, cook chives. Place in the garlic and broccoli and cook until soft as you stir occasionally. Stir in broth and fines herbes and cook for 6 more minutes.
3. Make 5 holes in the mixture until you are able to see the bottom of your pan. Crack an egg into each hole. Spread the cheese over the top and cook for 6 more minutes. Scatter the reserved ham over to serve.

Nutrition Info (Per Serving): Kcal 444; Fat: 35.3g, Net Carbs: 2.7g, Protein: 29.8g

Crostini with Avocado

Servings: 4

Cooking Time: 25 minutes

Ingredients

- 4 tbsp olive oil
- 2 avocados, chopped
- ¼ tsp garlic powder
- ¼ tsp onion powder
- 1 tbsp chopped parsley
- 1 lemon, zested and juiced
- 1 loaf zero carb bread, sliced
- 2 garlic cloves, halved
- 3 tbsp grated Parmesan
- 2 tbsp chopped toasted pecans

Directions:

1. In a bowl, using a fork, mix 2 tbsp of olive oil, avocado, garlic and onion powders, salt, pepper, parsley, zest, and juice until smooth; set aside. Heat a grill pan; rub both sides of the bread slices with garlic; brush with olive oil.

2. Grill on both sides in the heated pan until crispy and golden. Transfer crostini to a plate and spread generously with avocado mixture. Sprinkle with Parmesan cheese and some pecans. Drizzle with some olive oil and serve.

Nutrition Info (Per Serving): Cal 327; Net Carbs 3.9g; Fat 31g; Protein 3.6g

Speedy Beef Carpaccio

Servings: 4

Cooking Time: 10 minutes

Ingredients

- 1 tbsp olive oil
- ½ lemon, juiced
- Salt and black pepper to taste
- ¼ lb rare roast beef, sliced
- 1 ½ cups baby arugula
- ¼ cup grated Parmesan cheese

Directions:

1. In a bowl, whisk olive oil, lemon juice, salt, and pepper until well combined.
2. Spread the beef on a large Serves plate, top with arugula and drizzle the olive oil mixture on top.
3. Sprinkle with grated Parmesan cheese and serve.

Nutrition Info (Per Serving): Cal 106; Net Carbs 4.1g; Fat 5g; Protein 10g

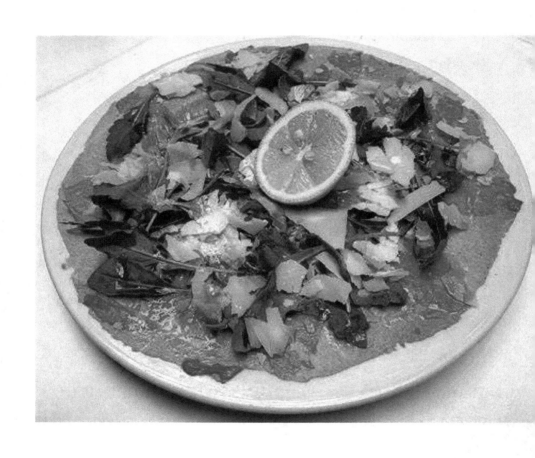

Cream Cheese & Caramelized Onion Dip

Servings: 4

Cooking Time: 30 minutes

Ingredients

- 2 tbsp butter
- 3 yellow onions, thinly sliced
- 1 tsp swerve sugar
- Salt to taste
- ¼ cup white wine
- 2 cups sour cream
- 8 oz cream cheese, softened
- ½ tbsp Worcestershire sauce

Directions:

1. Melt the butter into a skillet and add in onions, swerve sugar, and salt and cook with frequent stirring for -15 minutes.

2. Add in white wine, stir and allow sizzling out, 10 minutes.

3. In a Serves bowl, mix sour cream and cream cheese until well combined.

4. Add onions and Worcestershire sauce; stir well into the cream.

5. Serve with celery sticks.

Nutrition Info (Per Serving): Cal 383; Net Carbs 8.3g; Fat 34g; Protein 8g

Tuna and Spinach Salad

Servings: 2

Cooking Time: 0 minutes

Ingredients

- 4 oz tuna, packed in water
- 2 oz chopped spinach
- 1 tbsp grated mozzarella cheese
- 1/3 cup mayonnaise

Seasoning:

- ¼ tsp salt
- 1/8 tsp ground black pepper

Directions:

Take a bowl, add mayonnaise in it along with cheese, season with salt and black pepper and whisk until combined. Then add tuna and spinach, toss until mixed and serve.

Nutrition Info: 191 Calories; 16.6 g Fats; 9.6 g Protein; 0.8 g Net Carb; 0.2 g Fiber

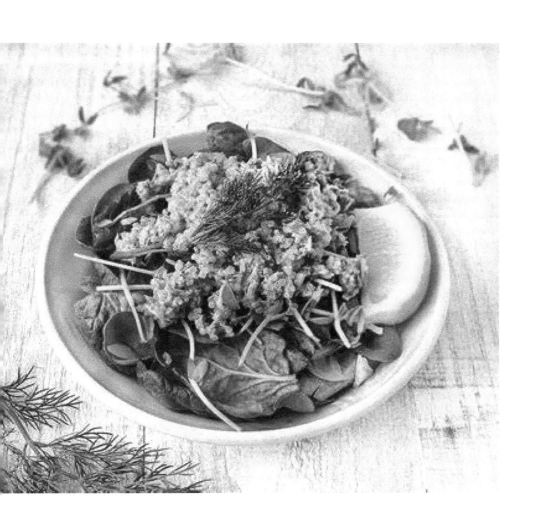

SOUP AND STEWS

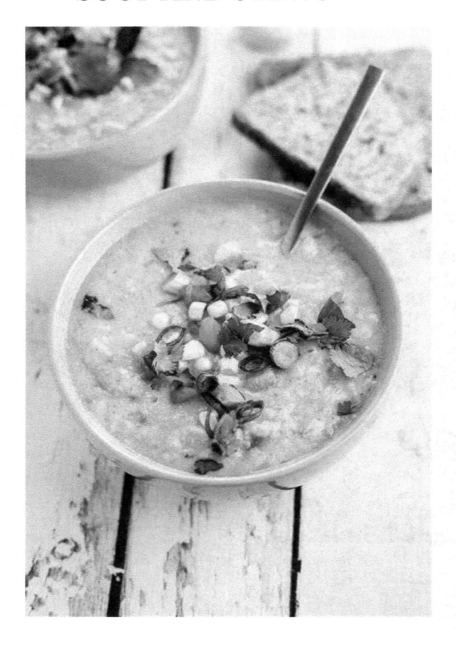

Cauliflower Kale Soup

Preparation Time: 10 minutes

Cooking Time: 50 minutes

Servings: 4

Ingredients:

- 4 cups cauliflower florets
- 6 cups vegetable stock
- 1 tbsp. garlic, minced
- 1/4 cup onion, chopped
- 6 oz kale, chopped
- 6 tbsp. olive oil
- Pepper Salt

Directions:

1. Preheat the oven to 425° F.
2. Spread cauliflower onto the baking tray and drizzle with two tablespoons of oil and season with pepper and salt.
3. Roast cauliflower in a preheated oven for 25 minutes. Remove from the oven and set aside.
4. In a bowl, toss kale with two tablespoons of oil and season with salt. Arrange kale onto the baking tray and bake at 300 F for 30 minutes. Toss halfway through.
5. Heat oil.

6. Add onion and sauté for 3-4 minutes. Add garlic and sauté for a minute. Add stock and roasted cauliflower and bring to boil.

7. Simmer it for 10 minutes.

8. Add kale and cook for 10 minutes more. Puree the soup until smooth.

9. Serve and enjoy.

Nutrition:

Calories: 287 Fat: 15.1g Fiber: 4.1g Carbohydrates: 3.1 g Protein: 5.8g

Healthy Celery Soup

Preparation Time: 10 minutes

Cooking Time: 20 minutes

Servings: 4

Ingredients:

- 3 cups celery, chopped
- 1 cup vegetable broth
- 5 oz cream cheese
- 1 1/2 tbsp. fresh basil, chopped
- 1/4 cup onion, chopped
- tbsp. garlic, chopped
- 1 tbsp. olive oil
- 1/4 tsp. pepper
- 1/2 tsp. salt

Directions:

1. Heat some oil.
2. Add celery, onion, and garlic to the saucepan and sauté for 4-5 minutes or until softened.
3. Add broth and bring to boil. Turn heat to low and simmer. Add basil and cream cheese and stir until cheese is melted. Season soup with pepper and salt.
4. Puree the soup until smooth. Serve and enjoy.

Nutrition:

Calories: 201 Fat: 5.4g Fiber: 8.1g Carbohydrates: 3.9 g Protein: 5.1g

Chinese Tofu Soup

Preparation Time: 5 minutes

Cooking Time: 5 minutes

Servings: 2

Ingredients:

- 2 cups chicken stock
- 1 tbsp. soy sauce, sugar-free
- 2 spring onions, sliced
- tsp. sesame oil, softened
- 2 eggs, beaten
- 1-inch piece ginger, grated
- Salt and black ground, to taste
- 1/2 pound extra-firm tofu, cubed
- A handful of fresh cilantro, chopped

Directions:

1. Boil in a pan over medium heat, soy sauce, chicken stock, and sesame oil. Place in eggs as you whisk to incorporate thoroughly.
2. Change heat to low and add salt, spring onions, black pepper, ginger; cook for 5 minutes.
3. Place in tofu and simmer for 1 to 2 minutes.
4. Divide into soup bowls and serve sprinkled with fresh cilantro.

Nutrition:

Calories: 178 Fat: 4.1g Fiber: 3.1g Carbohydrates: 0.4 g Protein: 5.5 g

Sausage & Cheese Beer Soup

Preparation Time: 15 minutes

Cooking Time: 8 hrs.

Servings: 4

Ingredients:

- tbsp. butter
- 1/2 cup celery, chopped
- 1/2 cup heavy cream
- 5 oz turkey sausage, sliced
- 1 small carrot, chopped
- 2 garlic cloves, minced
- 4 ounces cream cheese
- 1/2 tsp. red pepper flakes
- 1 cup beer of choice
- 3 cups beef stock
- 1 yellow onion, diced
- 1 cup cheddar cheese, grated
- Kosher salt and black pepper, to taste
- Fresh parsley, chopped, to garnish

Directions:

1. To the crockpot, add butter, beef stock, beer, turkey sausage, carrot, onion, garlic, celery, salt, red pepper flakes, and black pepper, and stir to combine.

2. Cook for 6 hrs. on low.

3. Then add in the cream, cheddar, and cream cheese, and cook for two more hours.

Nutrition:

Calories: 345 Fat: 10.4g Fiber: 9.4g Carbohydrates: 4.1 g Protein: 11.2g

Egg Drop Soup

Preparation Time: 5 minutes

Cooking Time: 10 minutes

Servings: 2

Ingredients:

- 4 cups chicken broth
- 1 teaspoon pink Himalayan sea salt
- 1/2 teaspoon ground ginger
- 1/2 teaspoon toasted sesame oil
- Pinch of ground white pepper
- 2 large eggs scallion

Directions:

1. In a medium saucepan, combine the broth, salt, ginger, sesame oil, and white pepper.
2. Cook over medium-high heat until the soup is boiling. In a small bowl, lightly beat the eggs.
3. Stirring the soup in a circular motion, slowly drizzle the beaten egg into the center of the vortex. When all the egg is mixed in, stop stirring.
4. Cook for an additional 2 minutes, until the egg is cooked through, then pour into 2 bowls, sprinkle with the scallions, and serve.

Nutrition:

Calories: 121 Fat: 5.1g Fiber: 2.9g Carbohydrates: 1.2 g Protein: 10g

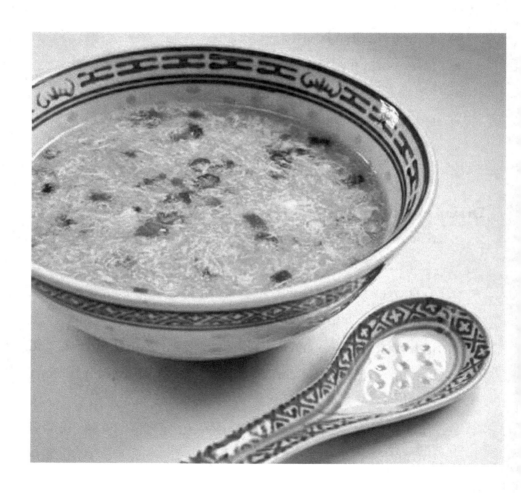

MAIN

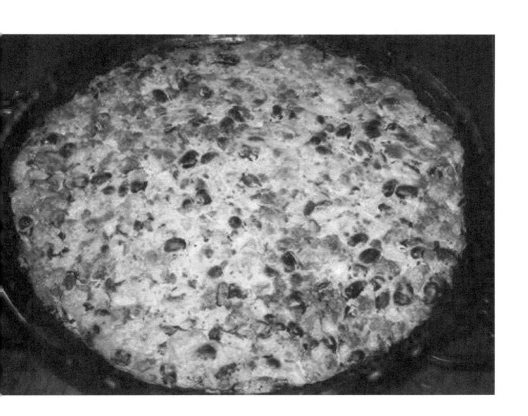

Chipotle Pizza with Cotija & Cilantro

Servings: 2

Cooking Time: 15 minutes

Ingredients

Pizza crust:

- 4 eggs, beaten
- ¼ cup sour cream
- 2 tbsp flaxseed meal
- 1 tsp chipotle pepper
- ¼ tsp cumin seeds, ground
- ½ tsp dried coriander leaves
- Salt to taste
- 1 tbsp olive oil

Topping:

- 2 tbsp tomato paste
- 2 ounces Cotija cheese, shredded
- Fresh chopped cilantro for garnish

Directions:

1. Mix all crust ingredients, except for the oil.
2. Set the pan over medium heat and warm ½ tablespoon oil. Ladle ½ of crust mixture into the pan and evenly spread out. Cook until the edges are set; then, flip the crust and

cook on the second side. Do the same process with the remaining crust mixture.

3. Warm the remaining ½ tablespoon of oil in the pan. Spread each pizza crust with tomato paste, then scatter over the cotija cheese. In batches, bake in the oven for 8-10 minutes at 425°F until all the cheese melts. Garnish with cilantro and serve.

Nutrition Info (Per Serving): Kcal 397, Fat: 31g, Net Carbs: 8.1g, Protein: 22G

Lemon Cauliflower "Couscous" with Halloumi

Preparation Time: 5 minutes

Cooking Time: 5 minutes

Servings: 2

Ingredients:

- 4 oz halloumi, sliced
- cauliflower head, cut into small florets
- 1/4 cup chopped cilantro
- 1/4 cup chopped parsley
- 1/4 cup chopped mint
- 1/2 lemon juiced
- Salt and black pepper to taste
- Sliced avocado to garnish

Directions:

1. Heat the pan and add oil
2. Add the halloumi and fry on both sides until golden brown, set aside. Turn the heat off.
3. Next, pour the cauliflower florets into a food processor and pulse until it crumbles and resembles couscous.
4. Transfer to a bowl and steam in the microwave for 2 minutes.
5. They should be slightly cooked, but crunchy.

6. Stir in the cilantro, parsley, mint, lemon juice, salt, and black pepper.

7. Garnish the couscous with avocado slices and serve with grilled halloumi and vegetable sauce.

Nutrition:

Calories: 312 Fat: 9.4g Fiber: 11.9g Carbohydrates: 1.2 g Protein: 8.5g

Black Bean Quiche

Servings: 6

Preparation Time: 10 minutes

Cooking Time: 35 minutes

Ingredients:

- Eggs - 5
- Egg whites - 5
- Water: 1/3 cup
- Salt: ½ teaspoon
- Ground pepper: ¼ teaspoon
- Black beans -low-sodium: 2/3 cup
- Tomato -chopped: ½ cup
- Jack cheese -grated: 3 oz.
- Cilantro: for garnish

Directions:

1. Whisk together the egg whites, eggs, salt, pepper, and water and pour the mixture into a pie dish greased with cooking spray.
2. Sprinkle the tomatoes, black beans, and cheese over the top and bake for 30-35 minutes at 375 degrees Fahrenheit until the egg sets at the center.
3. Leave to cool for 10 minutes.
4. Serve garnished with cilantro.

Nutrition Value:

141.7 Cal, 8.7 g total fat -1.4 g sat. fat, 172.5 mg chol., 402.8 mg sodium, 6.7 g carbs, 1.6g fiber, 10 g protein.

Kelp Noodles with Peanut Butter Sauce

Servings: 4

Preparation Time: 10 minutes

Cooking Time: 0 minutes

Ingredients:

- Kelp noodles: 1 bag

Sauce:

- Peanut butter: ½ cup
- White onion: 1
- Soy sauce: ¼ cup
- Lime juice: of 1 lime
- Garlic cloves: 3
- Red pepper flakes: 2 teaspoon

Directions:

1. Place all the sauce ingredients in a blender and blend until smooth.
2. Soak the kelp noodles in water and then drain.
3. Add ¼ of the sauce on top and serve.

Nutrition Value:

231 Cal, 16 g total fat, 7 g net carbs, 5g fiber, 7 g protein.

Cheesy Risotto

Servings: 4

Preparation Time: 15 minutes

Cooking Time: 5 minutes

Ingredients:

- Cauliflower -riced: 1
- Butter: ¼ cup
- White onion -chopped finely: 1
- Vegetable stock: 1 cup
- Dijon mustard: 1 teaspoon
- Cheddar cheese -shredded: 1 cup
- Parmesan cheese -grated: 1 cup
- Chives -chopped: 2 tablespoon
- Salt: to taste

Directions:

1. Melt some butter in a pan and sauté the onion in it until browned lightly.
2. Pour in the vegetable stock and cook for another 5 minutes.
3. Mix in the mustard and remove from the flame.
4. Season with salt and mix in the cheese.
5. Garnish with the chives.

Nutrition Value:

366 Cal, 28.8 g total fat -17.4 g sat. fat, 11.6 g carbs, 4g fiber, 17.4 g protein.

MEAT

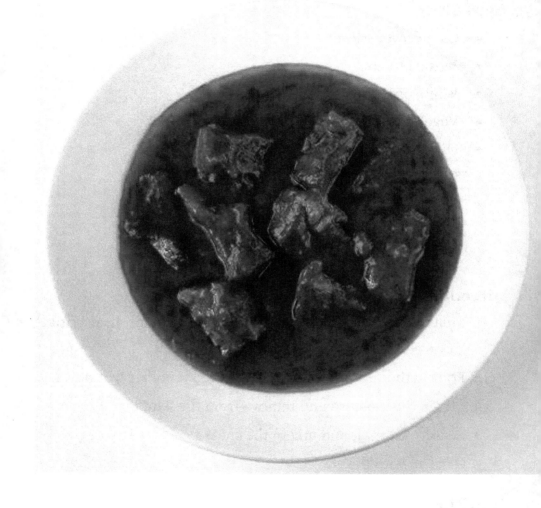

Dijon Pork Loin Roast

Servings: 6

Cooking Time: 30 minutes

Ingredients

- 3 lb boneless pork loin roast
- 5 cloves garlic, minced
- Salt and black pepper to taste
- 1 tbsp Dijon mustard
- 1 tsp dried basil
- 2 tsp garlic powder

Directions:

1. Preheat the oven to 400° F and place the pork in a baking dish. In a bowl, mix minced garlic, salt, pepper, mustard, basil, and garlic powder.
2. Rub the mixture onto pork. Drizzle with olive oil and bake for minutes or until cooked within and brown outside. Transfer onto a flat surface, and let cool for 5 minutes. Serve sliced with steamed greens.

Nutrition Info (Per Serving): Cal 311; Net Carbs 2g; Fat 9g; Protein 51g

Winter Beef Goulash

Servings: 6

Cooking Time: 3 Hours 10 minutes

Ingredients

- 1 tablespoon lard
- 2 pounds flank steak, cut against the grain into 6 pieces
- 2 bell peppers, chopped
- 1 onion, chopped
- 3 garlic cloves, finely chopped
- 1 celery stalk, chopped
- 1 fresh tomato, puréed
- 4 tablespoons tomato paste
- 2 bay laurels
- 1 teaspoon parsley flakes
- 1 thyme sprig
- 1 rosemary sprig
- Sea salt and ground black pepper, to taste
- 1 teaspoon red pepper flakes

Directions:

1. Melt the lard in a heavy-bottomed pot over medium-high heat. Once hot, sear the beef until no longer pink or about 5 minutes per side; reserve.

2. In the pan drippings, sauté the bell peppers, onions, garlic, and celery for 3 minutes or until just tender and fragrant.

3. Add the reserved beef back to the pot. Add in the remaining ingredients; gently stir to combine.

4. Cook in the preheated oven at 300 degrees F for 3 hours or until the meat is fork-tender and cooked through. Shred the meat with two forks and serve in individual bowls. Bon appétit!

Nutrition Info (Per Serving): 254 Calories; 9.8g Fat; 6.3g Carbs; 33.4g Protein; 1.2g Fiber

Spanish-style Scotch Fillet

Servings: 4

Cooking Time: 15 minutes

Ingredients

- 4 Scotch fillet steaks, about 1-inch thick
- 1 small bunch fresh flat-leaf parsley, chopped
- 1 tablespoon coconut aminos
- 1/2 cup Marsala wine
- 1 tablespoon sherry vinegar
- 4 cloves garlic, crushed
- Pink Himalayan salt and ground black pepper, to season
- 2 tablespoons butter, unsalted and softened
- 2 Spanish peppers, sliced
- 2 scallions, sliced
- 1/4 cup Spanish olives, pitted and halved

Directions:

1. Pat the Scotch fillet dry with paper towels and place in a ceramic dish. Add in the parsley, coconut aminos, wine, sherry vinegar, garlic, salt, and black pepper. Let it marinate in your refrigerator for 3 hours.

2. Melt the butter in a 1inch skillet over high heat until very hot.

3. Next, cook the steaks for 4 minutes. Flip them, add the peppers and scallions, and cook for a further 4 minutes for medium.

4. Serve with Spanish olives and enjoy!

Nutrition Info (Per Serving): 426 Calories; 21.8g Fat; 5.6g Carbs; 49g Protein; 1.4g Fiber

Sunday Pot Roast with Vegetable Mash

Servings: 5

Cooking Time: 1 Hour 25 minutes

Ingredients

- 1 teaspoon smoked paprika
- 1/2 teaspoon dried thyme
- 1/2 teaspoon dried rosemary
- Sea salt and cracked black pepper, to season
- 2 pounds beef chuck roast

Keto Vegetable Mash:

- 1/3 pound cauliflower florets
- 1/2 pound parsnips, chopped
- 2 tablespoons butter

Directions:

1. Season the chuck roast with paprika, thyme, rosemary, salt, and black pepper. Place on a tinfoil-lined baking pan.

2. Bake in the preheated oven at 370 degrees F for 40 minutes. Let it stand for 15 minutes before slicing and serving.

3. Meanwhile, place the cauliflower and parsnips in a deep saucepan; cover with water and cook until they have softened for 25 minutes.

4. Drain well. Fold in the butter and mash with a potato masher. Serve with the roast beef and enjoy!

Nutrition Info (Per Serving): 324 Calories; 15.1g Fat; 6.5g Carbs; 38.4g Protein; 2.8g Fiber

Beef Alfredo Squash Spaghetti

Servings: 4

Cooking Time: 1 Hour 20 minutes

Ingredients

- 2 medium spaghetti squashes, halved
- 2 tbsp olive oil
- 2 tbsp butter
- 1 lb ground beef
- ½ tsp garlic powder
- Salt and black pepper to taste
- 1 tsp arrowroot starch
- 1 ½ cups heavy cream
- A pinch of nutmeg
- 1/3 cup grated Parmesan
- 1/3 cup grated mozzarella

Directions:

1. Preheat oven to 375° F. Season the squash with olive oil, salt, and pepper. Place on a lined with foil baking dish and roast for 45 minutes. Let cool and shred the inner part of the noodles; set aside. Melt butter in a pot, add beef, garlic powder, salt, and pepper, and cook for minutes. Stir in arrowroot starch, heavy cream, and nutmeg.

2. Cook until the sauce thickens, 3 minutes. Spoon the sauce into the squashes and cover with Parmesan and mozzarella cheeses. Cook under the broiler for 3 minutes.

Nutrition Info (Per Serving): Cal 563; Net Carbs 4g; Fats 42g; Protein 36g

Bbq Pork Pizza with Goat Cheese

Servings: 4

Cooking Time: 30 minutes

Ingredients

- 1 low carb pizza bread
- Olive oil for brushing
- 1 cup grated Manchego cheese
- 2 cups leftover pulled pork
- ½ cup sugar-free BBQ sauce
- 1 cup crumbled goat cheese

Directions:

1. Preheat oven to 400° F and put pizza bread on a pizza pan.

2. Brush with olive oil and sprinkle the Manchego cheese all over.

3. Mix the pork with BBQ sauce and spread over the cheese. Drop goat cheese on top and bake for 25 minutes until the cheese has melted. Slice the pizza with a cutter and serve.

Gruyere Beef Burgers with Sweet Onion

Servings: 4

Cooking Time: 35 minutes

Ingredients

- 4 zero carb hamburger buns, halved
- 1 medium white onion, sliced
- 3 tbsp olive oil
- 2 tbsp balsamic vinegar
- 2 tbsp erythritol
- 1 lb ground beef
- Salt and black pepper to taste
- 4 slices Gruyere cheese
- Mayonnaise to serve

Directions:

1. Heat 2 tbsp of olive oil in a skillet and add the onion.
2. Sauté for minutes until golden brown and add erythritol, balsamic vinegar, and salt. Cook for 3 more minutes; set aside.
3. Make 4 patties out of the ground beef and season with salt and pepper.
4. Then, heat the remaining olive oil in a skillet and cook the patties for 4 minutes on each side. Place a Gruyere slice on each patty and top with the caramelized onions.

Put the patties with cheese and onions into two halves of the buns. Serve with mayonnaise.

Nutrition Info (Per Serving): Cal 487; Net Carbs 7.8g; Fat 32g; Protein 38g

Basil Prosciutto Pizza

Servings: 4

Cooking Time: 45 minutes

Ingredients

- 4 prosciutto slices, cut into thirds
- 2 cups grated mozzarella cheese
- 2 tbsp cream cheese, softened
- ½ cup almond flour
- 1 egg, beaten
- ⅓ cup tomato sauce
- ⅓ cup sliced mozzarella
- 6 fresh basil leaves, to serve

Directions:

1. Preheat oven to 390° F and line a pizza pan with parchment paper. Microwave mozzarella cheese and 2 tbsp of cream cheese for a minute. Mix in almond meal and egg.

2. Spread the mixture on the pizza pan and bake for 15 minutes; set aside. Spread the tomato sauce on the crust. Arrange the mozzarella slices on the sauce and then the prosciutto. Bake again for 15 minutes or until the cheese melts. Remove and top with the basil. Slice and serve.

Nutrition Info (Per Serving): Cal 160; Net Carbs 0.5g; Fats 6.2g; Protein 22g

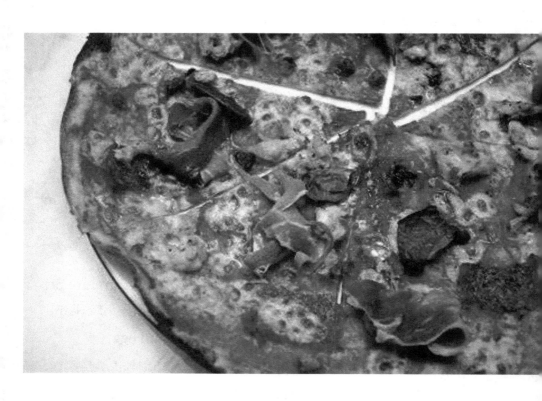

POULTRY

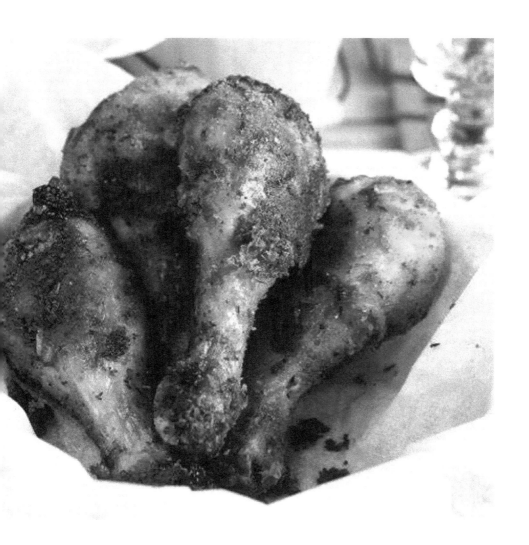

Acorn Squash Chicken Traybake

Servings: 4

Cooking Time: 60 minutes

Ingredients

- 2 lb chicken thighs
- 1 lb acorn squash, cubed
- ½ cup black olives, pitted
- ¼ cup olive oil
- 5 garlic cloves, sliced
- 1 tbsp dried oregano

Directions:

1. Set oven to 400 F. Places the chicken with the skin down in a greased baking dish.
2. Set garlic, olives and acorn squash around the chicken, then drizzle with oil. Spread pepper, salt, and thyme over the mixture. Bake for 45 minutes.

Nutrition Info (Per Serving): Cal: 411, Net Carbs: 5g, Fat: 15g, Protein: 31g

Celery & Radish Chicken Casserole

Servings: 4

Cooking Time: 50 minutes

Ingredients

- ½ lemon, juiced
- 3 tbsp basil pesto
- ¾ cup heavy cream
- ½ cup cream cheese softened
- 3 tbsp butter
- 2 lb chicken breasts, cubed
- 1 celery, chopped
- ¼ cup chopped tomatoes
- 1 lb radishes, sliced
- ½ cup shredded Pepper Jack

Directions:

1. Preheat oven to 400 F. In a bowl, combine lemon juice, pesto, heavy cream, cream cheese, salt, and pepper; set aside. Melt butter in a skillet, season the chicken with salt and pepper and cook in the fat until no longer pink. 8 minutes. Transfer to a greased casserole dish and spread the pesto mixture on top. Top with celery, tomatoes, and radishes.

2. Sprinkle cheese on top and bake for 30 minutes or until the cheese melts and golden brown on top. Remove from the oven, dish, and serve with braised green beans.

Nutrition Info (Per Serving): Cal 667; Net Carbs 0.8g; Fat 47g; Protein 51g

Chicken and Bacon Rolls

Servings: 4

Cooking Time: 45 minutes

Ingredients

- 1 tbsp fresh chives, chopped
- 8 ounces blue cheese
- 2 pounds chicken breasts, skinless, boneless, halved
- 12 bacon slices
- 2 tomatoes, chopped
- Salt and ground black pepper, to taste

Directions:

1. Set a pan over medium heat, place in the bacon, cook until halfway done, remove to a plate. In a bowl, stir together blue cheese, chives, tomatoes, pepper and salt.

2. Use a meat tenderizer to flatten the chicken breasts, season and lay blue cheese mixture on top. Roll them up, and wrap each in a bacon slice.

3. Place the wrapped chicken breasts in a greased baking dish, and roast in the oven at 370°F for 30 minutes. Serve on top of wilted kale.

Nutrition Info (Per Serving): Kcal 623, Fat 48g, Net Carbs 5g, Protein 38g

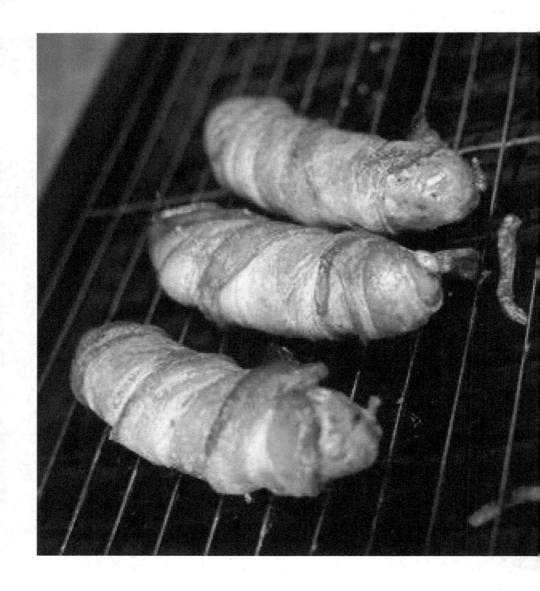

Parsley Chicken & Cauliflower Stir-fry

Servings: 4

Cooking Time: 30 minutes

Ingredients

- 1 large head cauliflower, cut into florets
- 2 tbsp olive oil
- 2 chicken breasts, sliced
- 1 red bell pepper, diced
- 1 yellow bell pepper, diced
- 3 tbsp chicken broth
- 2 tbsp chopped parsley

Directions:

1. Heat olive oil in a skillet and season chicken with salt and pepper; cook until brown on all sides, 8 minutes. Transfer to a plate.

2. Pour bell peppers into the pan and sauté until softened, 5 minutes. Add in cauliflower, broth, season to taste, and mix. Cover the pan and cook for 5 minutes or until cauliflower is tender.

3. Mix in chicken, parsley. Serve.

Nutrition Info (Per Serving): Cal 345; Net Carbs 3.5g; Fat 21g; Protein 32g

FISH

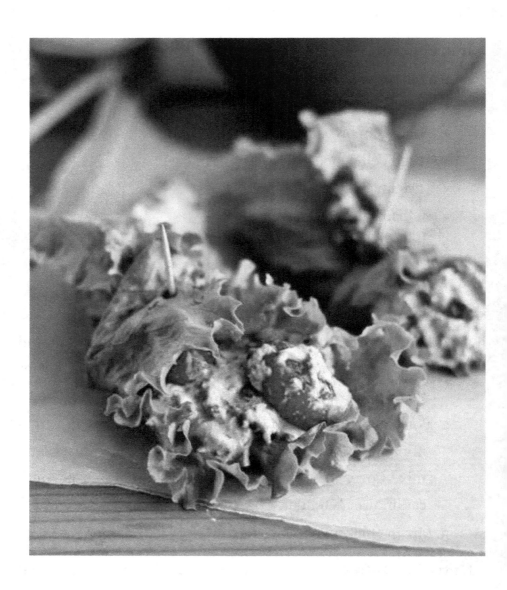

Greek Tuna Salad

Preparation Time: 10 minutes

Cooking Time: 0 minutes

Servings: 2

Ingredients:

- 3 cans tuna
- 1/4 small red onion, finely chopped
- 1 celery stalks, finely chopped
- 1/2 avocado, chopped
- tbsp. chopped fresh parsley
- 1 cup Greek yogurt
- tbsp. butter
- 2 tsp. Dijon Mustard
- 1/2 tbsp. vinegar
- Salt and black pepper to taste

Directions:

1. The ingredients listed must be added to a salad bowl and mix until well combined.
2. Serve afterward.

Nutrition:

Calories: 376 Fat: 10.4g Fiber: 11.9g Carbohydrates: 3.9 g Protein: 18.4g

Blackened Salmon with Avocado Salsa

Preparation Time: 15 minutes

Cooking Time: 10 minutes

Servings: 4

Ingredients:

- 1 tbsp. extra virgin olive oil
- 4 filets of salmon (about 6 oz. each)
- 4 tsp. Cajun seasoning
- 2 med. avocados, diced
- 1 c. cucumber, diced
- 1/4 c. red onion, diced
- 1 tbsp. parsley, chopped
- 1 tbsp. lime juice
- Sea salt & pepper, to taste

Directions:

1. The oil must be heated in a skillet.
2. Rub the Cajun seasoning into the fillets, then lay them into the bottom of the skillet once it's hot enough.
3. Cook until a dark crust forms, then flip and repeat.
4. In a medium mixing bowl, combine all the ingredients for the salsa and set aside.
5. Plate the fillets and top with 1/4 of the salsa yielded. Enjoy!

Nutrition:

Calories: 425 Fat: 15.8g Fiber: 19.2g Carbohydrates: 4.1 g Protein: 11/8g

Tangy Coconut Cod

Preparation Time: 10 minutes

Cooking Time: 10 minutes

Servings: 2

Ingredients:

- 1/3 c. coconut flour
- 1/2 tsp. cayenne pepper
- 1 egg, beaten
- 1 lime
- 1 tsp. crushed red pepper flakes
- 1 tsp. garlic powder
- 12 oz. cod fillets
- Sea salt & pepper, to taste

Directions:

1. Let the oven preheat to 400° F/175° C, then line a baking sheet with non-stick foil.

2. Place the flour in a shallow dish (a plate works fine) and drag the fillets of cod through the beaten egg. Dredge the cod in the coconut flour, then lay it on the baking sheet.

3. Sprinkle the fillet's top with the seasoning and lime juice.

4. Bake the cod for about 10 to 12 minutes until the fillets are flaky. Serve immediately!

Nutrition:

Calories: 318 Fat: 12.1g Fiber: 15.1g Carbohydrates: 4.1 g Protein: 19.5g

Fish Taco Bowl

Preparation Time: 10 minutes

Cooking Time: 15 minutes

Servings: 2

Ingredients:

- 2 (5-ounce) tilapia fillets
- 1 tablespoon olive oil
- 4 teaspoons Tajin seasoning salt, divided
- 2 cups pre-sliced coleslaw cabbage mix
- 1 tablespoon avocado mayo
- 1 tsp. hot sauce
- 1 avocado, mashed
- Pink Himalayan salt
- Freshly ground black pepper

Directions:

1. Preheat the oven to 425° F. The baking sheet must be lined with a baking mat.
2. Rub the tilapia with olive oil, and then coat it with two teaspoons of Tajín seasoning salt.
3. Place the fish in the prepared pan.
4. Let the tilapia bake for 15 minutes, or until the fish is opaque when you pierce it with a fork.

5. Meanwhile, in a medium bowl, gently mix to combine the coleslaw and the mayo sauce.

6. You don't want the cabbage super wet, just enough to dress it.

7. Add the mashed avocado and the remaining two teaspoons of Tajín seasoning salt to the coleslaw, and season with pink Himalayan salt and pepper.

8. Divide the salad between two bowls.

9. Shred fish into tiny pieces, and add them to the bowls. Top the fish with a drizzle of mayo sauce and serve.

Nutrition:

Calories: 231 Fat: 12.1g Fiber: 10.3g Carbohydrates: 2.1 g Protein: 17.3g

Scallops with Creamy Bacon Sauce

Preparation Time: 5 minutes

Cooking Time: 20 minutes

Servings: 2

Ingredients:

- 4 bacon slices
- 1 cup heavy (whipping) cream
- 1 tablespoon butter
- 1/4 cup grated Parmesan cheese
- Pink Himalayan salt
- Freshly ground black pepper
- 1 tablespoon ghee
- 8 large sea scallops, rinsed and patted dry

Directions:

1. Cook the bacon.

2. Lower the heat to medium. Add the butter, cream, and Parmesan cheese to the bacon grease and season with a pinch of pink Himalayan salt and pepper.

3. Lower the heat down, then stir constantly until the sauce thickens and is reduced by 50 percent, about 10 minutes.

4. In another skillet, heat the ghee until sizzling.

5. Season the scallops with pink Himalayan salt and pepper, and add them to the skillet—Cook for just 1 minute per side.

6. Do not crowd the scallops; if your pan isn't large enough, cook them in two batches.

7. You want the scallops golden on each side. Transfer the scallops to a paper towel-lined plate.

8. Divide the cream sauce between two plates, crumble the bacon on top of the cream sauce, and top with four scallops. Serve immediately.

Nutrition:

Calories: 311 Fat: 14.1g Fiber: 10.3g Carbohydrates: 1.2 g Protein: 17.7g

Parmesan-Garlic Salmon with Asparagus

Preparation Time: 10 minutes

Cooking Time: 15 minutes

Servings: 2

Ingredients:

- 2 (6-ounce) salmon fillets, skin on
- Pink Himalayan salt
- Freshly ground black pepper
- 1-pound fresh asparagus ends snapped off
- 3 tablespoons butter
- 2 garlic cloves, minced
- 1/4 cup grated Parmesan cheese

Directions:

1. Oven: 400° F.
2. Pat the salmon dry and season both sides with pink Himalayan salt and pepper.
3. Put the salmon, and arrange the asparagus around the salmon.
4. Melt the butter. Add the minced garlic and stir until the garlic just begins to brown about 3 minutes.
5. Drizzle the garlic-butter sauce over the salmon and asparagus, and top both with the Parmesan cheese.

6. Bake until the salmon is cooked and the asparagus is crisp-tender, about 12 minutes. You can switch the oven to broil at the end of cooking time to char the asparagus.

7. Serve hot.

Nutrition:

Calories: 476 Fat: 14.1g Fiber: 10.5g Carbohydrates: 3.1 g Protein: 19.9g

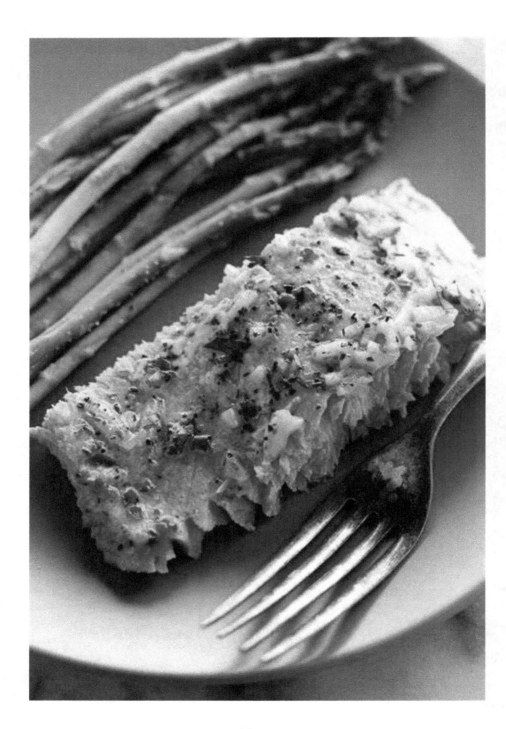

Spicy Shrimp Skewers

Preparation Time: 5 minutes

Cooking Time: 3-9 minutes

Servings: 4

Ingredients:

- 2 tbsp. Paprika
- 1/2 tbsp. Onion powder
- 1/2 tbsp. dried thyme, crushed
- 1-pound shrimp, peeled and deveined
- 2 tbsp. Olive oil
- 1/2 tbsp. Red chili powder
- 1/2 tbsp. Garlic powder
- 1/2 tbsp. dried oregano, crushed
- 2 zucchinis, cut into 1/2-inch cubes

Directions:

1. Preheat the grill to medium-high heat. In a bowl, mix spices and dried herbs.
2. In a large bowl, add shrimp, zucchini, oil, and seasoning and toss to coat well.
3. Thread shrimp and zucchini onto pre-soaked skewers.
4. Grill the skewers for about 6-8 minutes, flipping occasionally. Serve hot.

Nutrition:

Calories: 261 Fat: 9.4g Fiber: 10.1g Carbohydrates: 3.2 g Protein: 4.1g

VEGETABLES

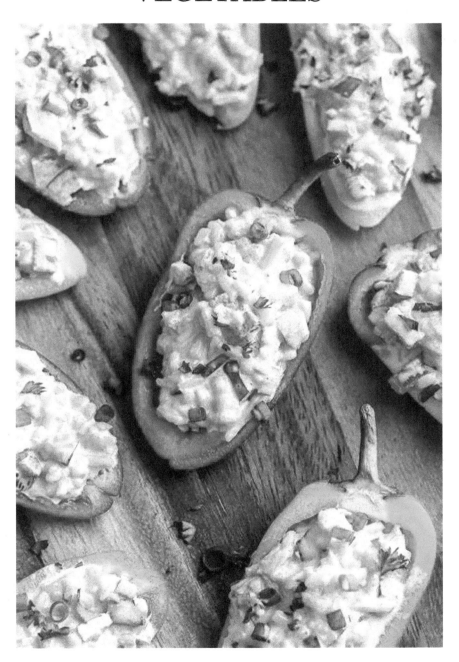

Delicious Asian Lunch Salad

Servings: 4

Cooking Time: 15 minutes

Ingredients

- 1 pound beef, ground
- 1 tablespoon sriracha
- 2 tablespoons coconut aminos
- 2 garlic cloves, minced
- 10 ounces coleslaw mix
- 2 tablespoon sesame seed oil
- Salt and black pepper to the taste
- 1 teaspoon apple cider vinegar
- 1 teaspoon sesame seeds
- 1 green onion stalk, chopped

Directions:

1. Heat up a pan. Oil over medium heat, add garlic and brown for a minute.
2. Add beef, stir and cook for 10 minutes.
3. Add coleslaw mix, toss to coat and cook for 1minute.
4. Add vinegar, sriracha, coconut aminos, salt and pepper, stir and cook for minutes more.
5. Add green onions and sesame seeds, toss to coat, divide into bowls and serve for lunch.
6. Enjoy!

Nutrition Info:

Calories 350, fat 23, fiber 6, carbs 3, protein 20

Rosemary Cheese Chips with Guacamole

Servings: 4

Cooking Time: 20 minutes

- **Ingredients**
- 1 tbsp rosemary
- 1 cup Grana Padano, grated
- ¼ tsp sweet paprika
- ¼ tsp garlic powder
- 2 avocados, pitted and scooped
- 1 tomato, chopped

Directions:

1. Preheat oven to 350° F and line a baking sheet with parchment paper. Mix Grana Padano cheese, paprika, rosemary, and garlic powder evenly.

2. Spoon 6-8 teaspoons on the baking sheet, creating spaces between each mound.; flatten mounds. Bake for 5 minutes, cool, and remove to a plate.

3. To make the guacamole, mash avocado with a fork in a bowl, add in tomato and continue to mash until mostly smooth. Season with salt. Serve crackers with guacamole.

Nutrition Info (Per Serving): Cal 229; Net Carbs 2g; Fat 20g; Protein 10g

Mini Stuffed Peppers

Servings: 5

Cooking Time: 15 minutes

Ingredients

- 2 teaspoons olive oil
- 1 teaspoon mustard seeds
- 5 ounces ground turkey
- Salt and ground black pepper, to taste
- 10 mini bell peppers, cut in half lengthwise, stems and seeds removed
- 2 ounces garlic and herb seasoned chevre goat cheese, crumbled

Directions:

1. Heat the oil in a skillet over medium-high heat. Once hot, cook mustard seeds with ground turkey until the turkey is no longer pink. Crumble with a fork. Season with salt and black pepper.

2. Lay the pepper halves cut-side-up on a parchment-lined baking sheet. Spoon the meat mixture into the center of each pepper half.

3. Top each pepper with cheese. Bake in the preheated oven at 400 degrees F for 10 minutes. Bon appétit!

Nutrition Info (Per Serving): 198 Calories; 17.2g Fat; 3g Carbs; 0.9g Fiber; 7.8g Protein;

Golden Cheese Crisps

Servings: 4

Cooking Time: 10 minutes

Ingredients

- 1 cup Edam cheese
- 1 cup provolone cheese
- 1/3 teaspoon dried oregano
- 1/3 teaspoon dried rosemary
- ½ teaspoon garlic powder
- 1/3 teaspoon dried basil

Directions:

1. Preheat your oven to 390° F.

2. In a small bowl, mix the dried oregano, rosemary, basil, and garlic powder. Set aside. Combine the Edam cheese and provolone cheese in another medium bowl.

3. Line a large baking dish with parchment paper, place tablespoon-sized stacks of the cheese mixture on the baking dish. Sprinkle with the dry seasonings mixture and bake for 6-7 minutes.

4. Let cool for a few minutes and enjoy.

Nutrition Info (Per Serving): 296 Calories; 22.7g Fat; 1.8g Carbs; 0.1g Fiber; 22g Protein

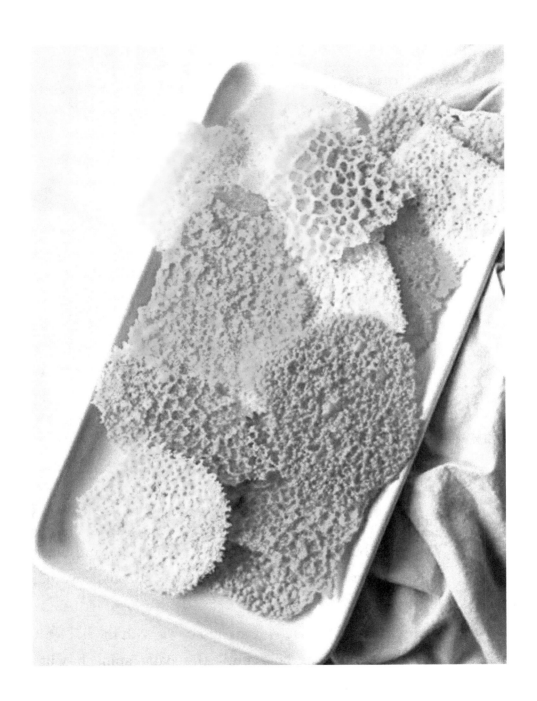

Butternut Squash & Spinach Stew

Servings: 4

Cooking Time: 35 minutes

Ingredients

- 2 tablespoons olive oil
- 1 Spanish onion, peeled and diced
- 1 garlic clove, minced
- 1/2 pound butternut squash, diced
- 1 celery stalk, chopped
- 3 cups vegetable broth
- Kosher salt and freshly cracked black pepper, to taste
- 4 cups baby spinach
- 4 tablespoons sour cream

Directions:

1. Heat the olive oil in a soup pot over a moderate flame. Now, sauté the Spanish onion until tender and translucent.
2. Then, cook the garlic until just tender and aromatic.
3. Stir in the butternut squash, celery, broth, salt, and black pepper. Turn the heat to simmer and let it cook, covered, for minutes.
4. Fold in the baby spinach leaves and cover with the lid; let it sit in the residual heat until the baby spinach wilts completely. Serve dolloped with cold sour cream. Enjoy!

Nutrition Info (Per Serving): 148 Calories; 11.5g Fat; 6.8g Carbs; 2.5g Protein; 2.3g Fiber

Italian-style Asparagus with Cheese

Servings: 2

Cooking Time: 10 minutes

Ingredients

- 1/2 pound asparagus spears, trimmed, cut into bite-sized pieces
- 1 teaspoon Italian spice blend
- 1/2 tablespoon lemon juice
- 1 tablespoon extra-virgin olive oil
- 4 tablespoons Romano cheese, freshly grated

Directions:

1. Bring a saucepan of lightly salted water to a boil. Turn the heat to medium-low. Add the asparagus spears and cook for approximately 3 minutes. Drain and transfer to a serving bowl.

2. Add the Italian spice blend, lemon juice, and extra-virgin olive oil; toss until well coated.

3. Top with Romano cheese and serve immediately. Bon appétit!

Nutrition Info (Per Serving): 193 Calories; 14.1g Fat; 5.6g Carbs; 11.5g Protein; 2.4g Fiber

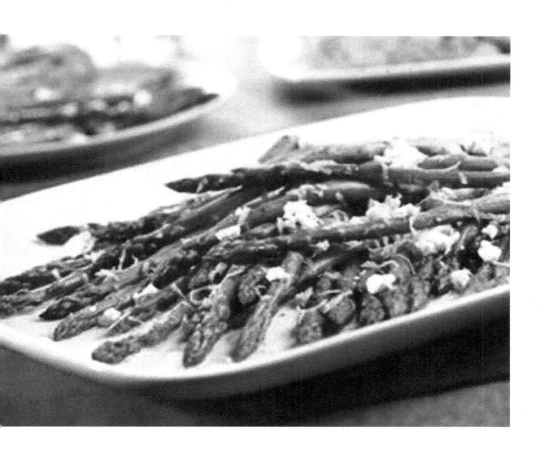

Cauliflower and Cashew Nuts Indian Style

Preparation Time: 15 minutes

Cooking Time: 35 minutes

Servings: 3

Ingredients:

- 1 very large cauliflower: florets and stems chopped into medium pieces
- 3 tbsp. coconut oil
- 1 tsp. cumin seeds
- 1 small handful of curry leaves
- ½ tsp. fennel seeds
- 4 cardamom pods
- ½ white onion - finely chopped
- 5 cloves of garlic: minced
- 1-inch piece of ginger: minced
- 2 medium tomatoes –chopped
- ½ cup Cashew nuts
- 1 tbsp. coriander powder
- ½ tsp. turmeric powder
- ½ tsp. Garam Masala
- ½ cup of coconut cream
- ¼ cup of water
- Fresh Coriander: roughly chopped
- Salt & Pepper

Directions:

1. Heat the coconut oil in a large pot over medium heat.

2. Add cardamom pods, cumin, and fennel seeds.

3. When the seeds start splattering, add the onion and curry leaves.

4. Fry for a couple of minutes, then adds a pinch of salt, stir and keep cooking until the onion is translucent - approximately 5 minutes.

5. Add ginger and garlic and cook for another 2-3 minutes.

6. Add the spices and stir-fry for a couple of minutes, until fragrant.

7. Add the chopped tomatoes, stir and cook for 5 minutes.

8. When the mixture becomes mushy, add the cauliflower and cashew nuts. Stir well together.

9. Add the water and coconut cream. Mix well.

10. Bring to boil. Cover the pot and cook over medium heat for about 12-15 minutes depending on how tender you like your cauliflower.

11. Remove from the heat. Add salt and pepper to taste, fresh coriander and stir.

12. Cover and let it rest for 5 minutes before serving.

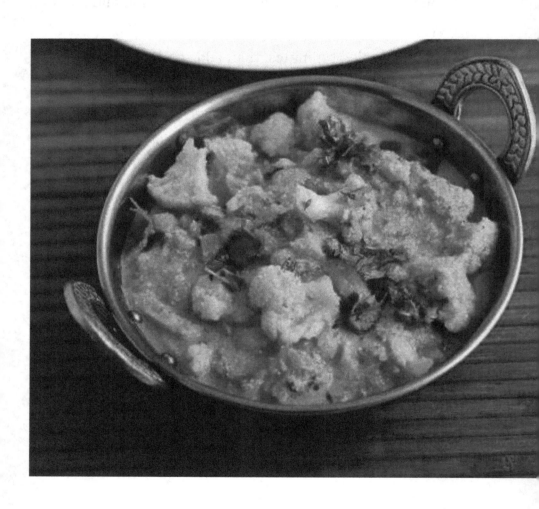

DESSERT

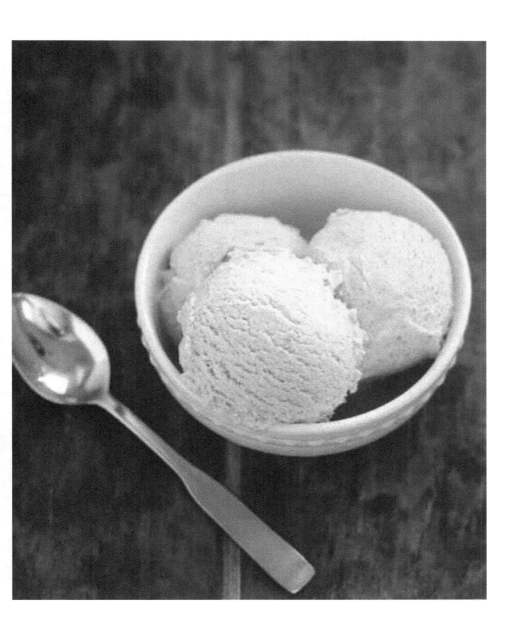

Strawberry and Basil Lemonade

Servings: 4

Cooking Time: 3 minutes

Ingredients

- 4 cups of water
- 12 strawberries, leaves removed
- 1 cup fresh lemon juice
- ⅓ cup fresh basil
- ¾ cup swerve
- Crushed Ice
- Halved strawberries to garnish
- Basil leaves to garnish

Directions:

1. Spoon some ice into 4 serving glasses and set aside. In a pitcher, add the water, strawberries, lemon juice, basil, and swerve. Insert the blender and process the ingredients for 30 seconds.

2. The mixture should be pink and the basil finely chopped. Adjust the taste and add the ice to the glasses. Drop strawberry halves and some basil in each glass and serve immediately.

Nutrition Info (Per Serving): Kcal 66, Fat 0.1g, Net Carbs 5.8g, Protein 0.7g

Cinnamon Cream

Servings: 4

Cooking Time: 10 minutes

Ingredients

- 2 tablespoons swerve
- 1 cup of coconut milk
- 1 cup heavy cream
- 1 tablespoon cinnamon powder
- ¼ teaspoon ginger, ground

Directions:

1. In a bowl, combine the cream with the milk and the other ingredients, whisk well, transfer to a pot, heat up over medium heat for minutes and divide into bowls.

2. Keep in the fridge for hours before serving.

Nutrition Info: calories 244, fat 25.4, fiber 1.3, carbs 5.2, protein 2

Lemon Custard

Servings: 4

Cooking Time: 40 minutes

Ingredients

- 1 cup heavy cream
- 2/3 cup swerve sugar
- 3 large lemons, juiced
- A pinch of cinnamon powder
- 6 egg yolks
- 2 tsp vanilla extract

Directions:

1. Heat heavy cream over medium heat and whisk in half of the swerving until well combined. Turn off the heat and let warm. In a separate bowl, whisk lemon juice, cinnamon, yolks, and vanilla.

2. Mix the egg mixture into the heavy cream one, turn on the heat and cook for minutes, whisking until thickened without boiling the mixture.

3. Remove from heat and pour into 4 ramekins. Chill for4 hours and serve.

Nutrition Info (Per Serving): Cal 225; Net Carbs 4.1g; Fat 18g; Protein 10g

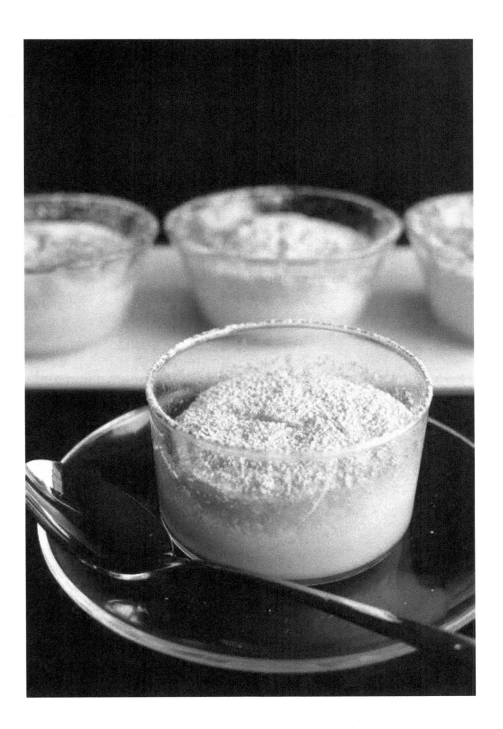

Avocado and Watermelon Salad

Servings: 4

Cooking Time: 0 minutes

Ingredients

- 2 avocados pitted, peeled and cubed
- 2 cups watermelon, peeled and cubed
- 1 tablespoon stevia
- 1 cup heavy cream
- 1 tablespoon mint, chopped

Directions:

1. In a bowl, combine the avocados with the watermelon and the other ingredients, toss and keep in the fridge for 2 hours before serving.

Nutrition Info: calories 271, fat 24.5, fiber 6.3, carbs 14.1, protein 2.8

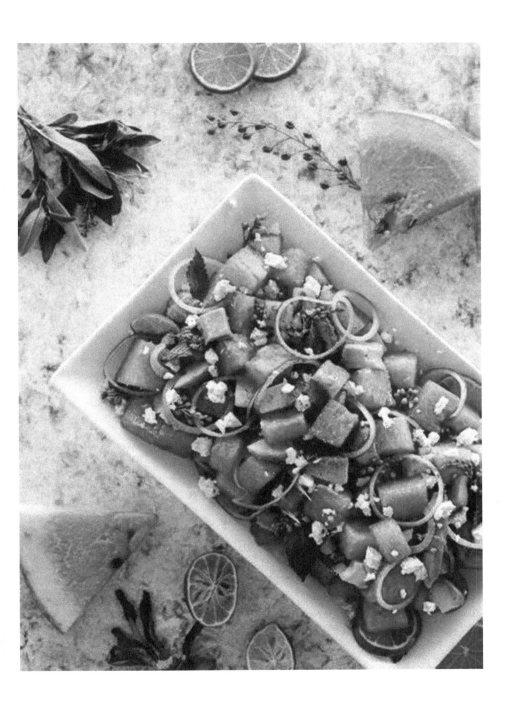

Mocha Mousse Cups

Servings: 4

Cooking Time: 10 minutes

Ingredients

- 8 oz cream cheese, softened
- 3 tbsp sour cream
- 2 tbsp butter, softened
- 1 ½ tsp vanilla extract
- 1/3 cup erythritol
- 3 tsp instant coffee powder
- ¼ cup of cocoa powder
- 2/3 cup heavy whipping cream
- 1 ½ tsp swerve sugar
- ½ tsp vanilla extract

Directions:

1. In a bowl using an electric hand mixer, beat cream cheese, sour cream, and butter until smooth. Mix in vanilla, erythritol, coffee, and cocoa powders until incorporated. In a separate bowl, beat whipping cream until soft peaks form. Mix in swerve sugar and vanilla until well combined.

2. Fold 1/3 of the whipped cream mixture into the cream cheese mixture to lighten. Fold in the remaining mixture until well incorporated. Spoon into dessert cups and serve.

Nutrition Info (Per Serving): Cal 308; Net Carbs 4g; Fat 30g; Protein 5g

Chocolate Ice Pops

Servings: 8

Cooking Time: 10 minutes

Ingredients

- 1 3/4 cups plain yogurt
- 4 tablespoons full-fat milk
- 5 tablespoons cocoa powder
- 1/2 teaspoon pure vanilla essence
- 3/4 cup Swerve

Directions:

1. Place all ingredients in a bowl of your food processor.

2. Pour into popsicle molds and freeze. Bon appétit!

Nutrition Info (Per Serving): 58 Calories; 2.6g Fat; 5.5g Carbs; 3.1g Protein; 1.2g Fiber